How to live a normal life when you are Bipolar

Table of Contents

Dedication's Page

This book is dedicated to all of the medical professionals who assist people when they are Bipolar

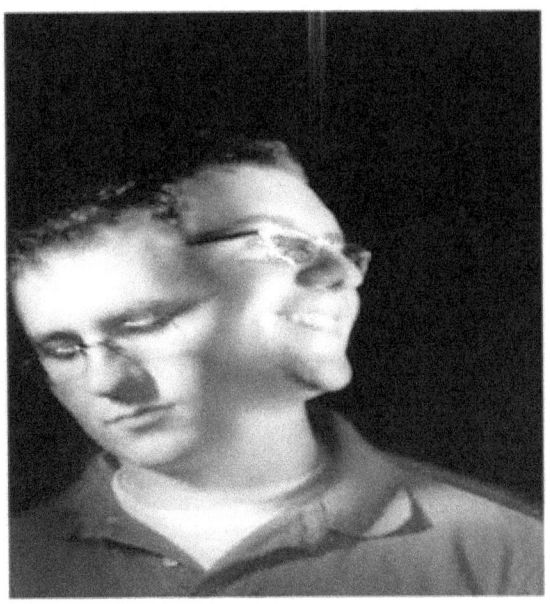

Courtesy of pschclasses2.wikispaces.com

A brief overview of a Bipolar Disorder

People with a Bipolar Disorder may have severe mood swings as well as

mania.

This terminology used to be called Manic Depression Disorder.

This medical condition is very serious and can cause suicidal tendencies,

all sorts of risky behavior but the good news is that it can be treated

with therapy and medication.

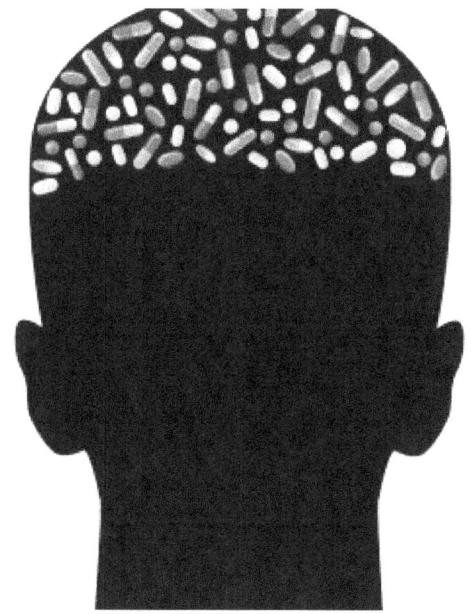

Photo courtesy of Practical Pedal

Some common symptoms and types of Bipolar Disorders

Bipolar Depression is a very complex disorder.

There are many different symptoms for a bipolar medical condition.

There are also several types of Bipolar Disorders that sometimes people

may not know about or understand.

The primary symptom of someone that has a bipolar disorder would be

the unpredictable and dramatic mood swings.

Some types of bipolar disorder can range from mild to severe as well.

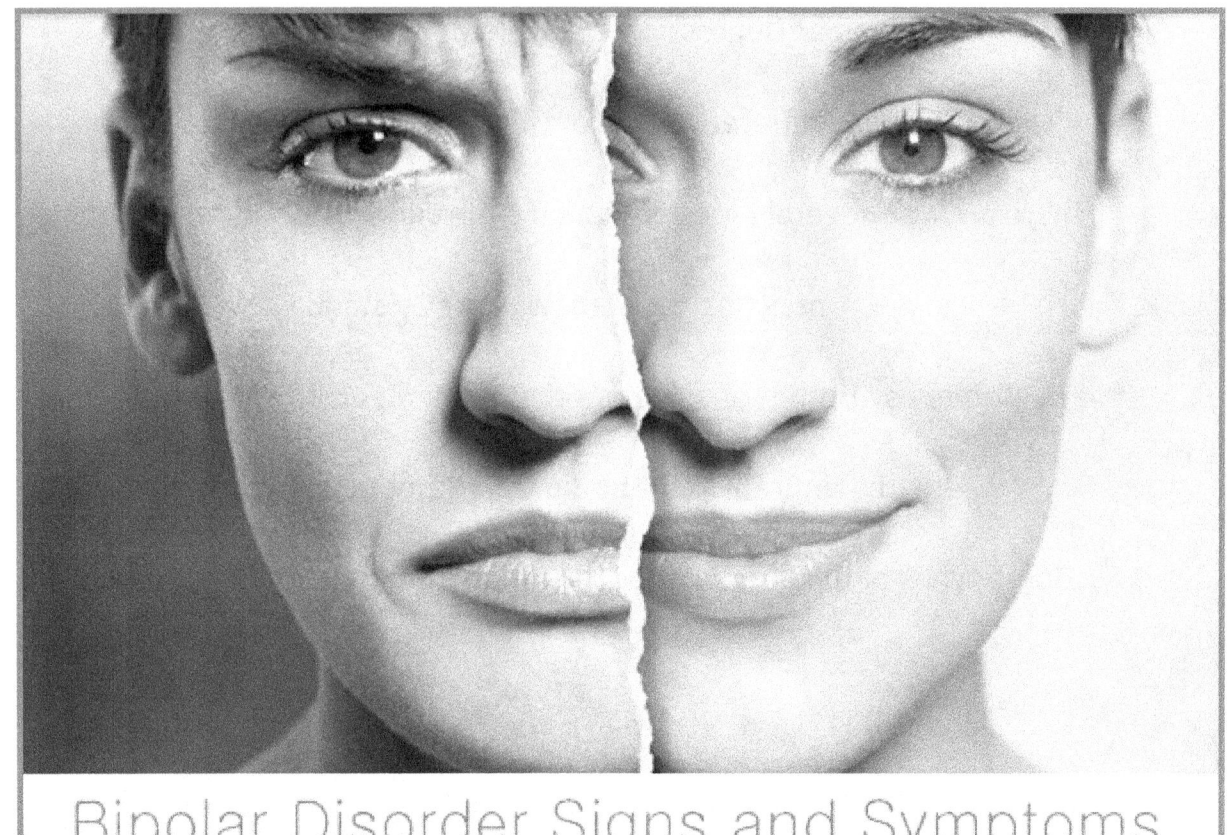

Bipolar Disorder Signs and Symptoms

Photo is the courtesy of Practical Pedal

Some symptoms of Bipolar Disorders

The Bipolar symptoms are unpredictable and dramatic mood swings.

Some of the Mania symptoms may include:

❖ Irritability

❖ Excessive happiness

❖ Less need for sleep

❖ Increased energy and high sex drive

❖ Racing thoughts and striving for unattainable goals

Some Depression symptoms of a Bipolar Disorder may be:

❖ Irritability

❖ Sadness

❖ Loss of Energy and A need for more sleep

❖ Anxiety

❖ Suicidal thoughts

Some types of Bipolar Disorders

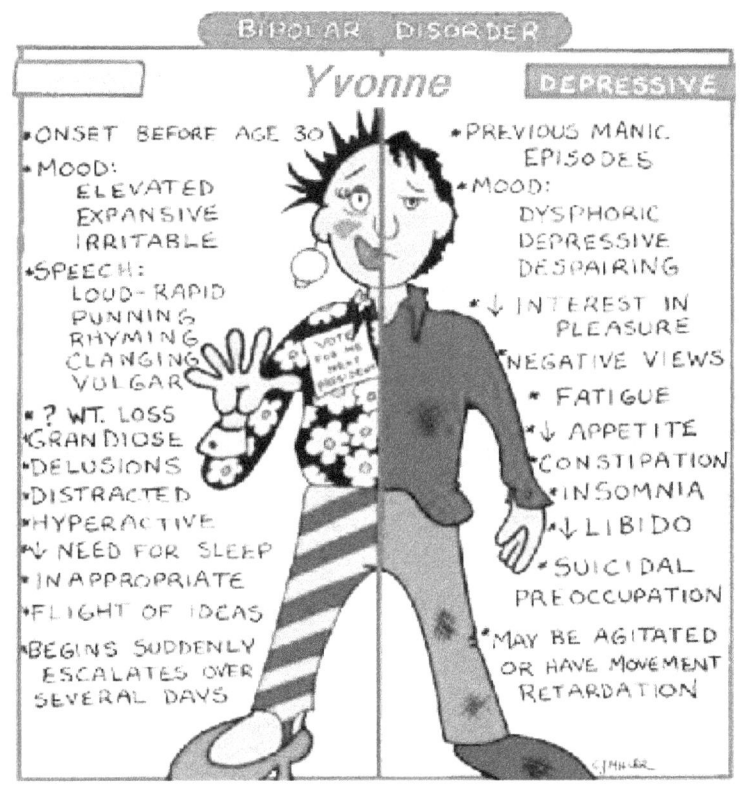

Photo is the courtesy of Wikispaces.com

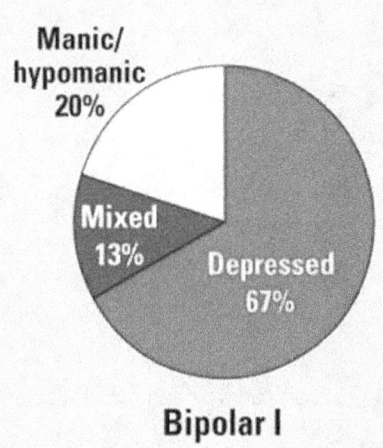

Bipolar I

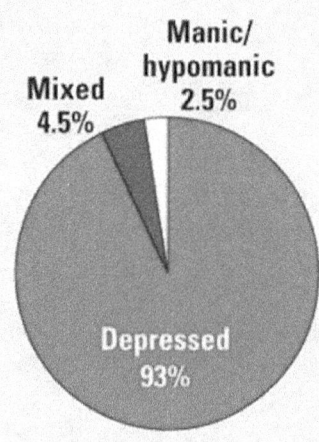

Bipolar II

- Patients with bipolar I experienced mood symptoms 47.3% of the time

- Patients with bipolar II experienced mood symptoms 54% of the time

- Depression was 3.4-fold more frequent than mania

- Depression was 37-fold more frequent than mania

Courtesy of Practice Pedal

Bipolar I

A person who has been diagnosed with Bipolar I has suffered at least one medical episode of an elevated mood swing and with this happening, this is accompanied by behavior that is considered abnormal and disrupts their life in some type of way.

Bipolar II

This type of Bipolar Disorder is very similar to the Bipolar I. An individual that may have this disorder always have "ups and downs" that may cycle between low and high all over time. The "up" stage never reaches full mania however.

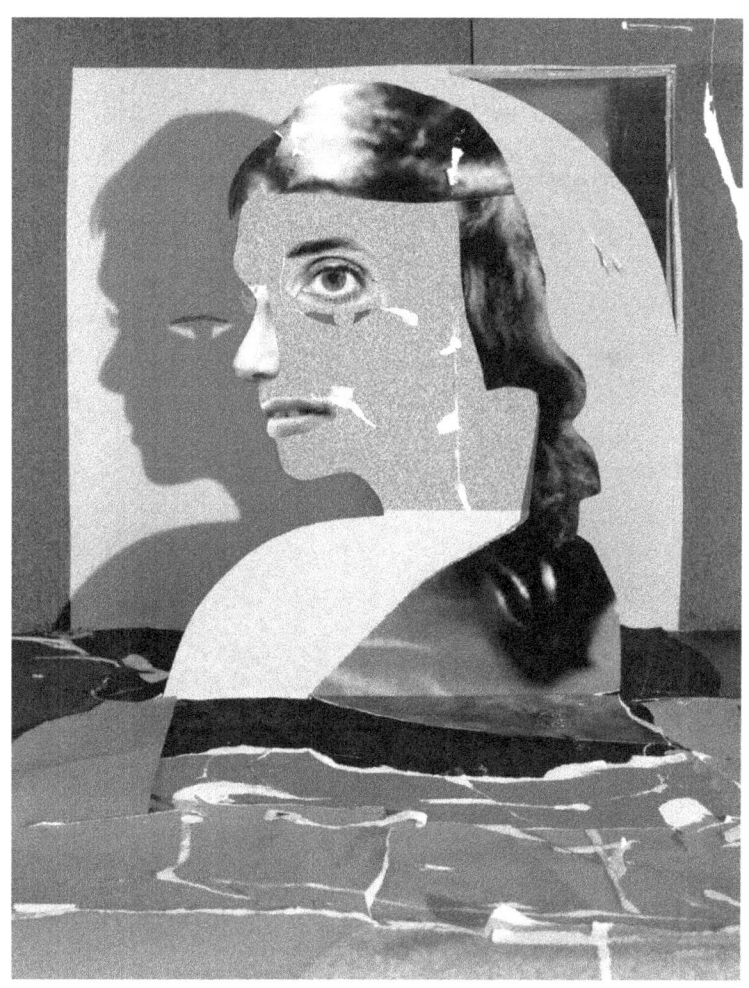

Photo courtesy of Practice Pedal

Some people may not know that there may be several types of Bipolar Disorders.

All of these types of Bipolar Disorders contain Depression and Mania to some degree.

Rapid Cycling

An individual that has rapid cycling bipolar disorder may have four to five episodes of depression or mania all in one year. People with rapid cycling calculate approximately 10-20% of the population.

Mixed Bipolar Disorders

A person that may be diagnosed with a Mixed Bipolar Disorder may have mood swings that may be elevated or depressed all over a period of time. A person that may have this type of medical condition may medical experiences with depression and mania in a rapid cycle or simultaneously.

Cyclothymia Bipolar Disorder

A person that may suffer from cyclothymia (cyclothymic disorder) bipolar disorder may suffer from only a mild mood disorder. An individual that may suffer from this medical condition can have milder symptoms than an individual suffering from a full-blown bipolar disorder.

Some Bipolar Complications and Warning Signs

People that suffer from any type of Bipolar Disorders may attempt self-harm of some sort. They may mutilate themselves by cutting or burning their bodies. They usually do this so that they may cope with any negative emotions that they may have about anger, frustrations or anxiety or some kind.

When an individual's medical condition follows a unique classical pattern, diagnosing them with a bipolar disorder is usually simple. Bipolar disorders can be very sneaky however. Some people's symptoms can defy the basic manic-depressive sequence.

People must remember that suicide is a very real threat when people are diagnosed with a bipolar disorder of some sort. Roughly, 10-15% of bipolar individuals may attempt suicide but with the proper treatments, the risks can be lowered.

Bipolar Diagnosis and Testing Procedures

Physicians can now diagnose individuals a lot easier. The medical understanding of a bipolar disorder can be by a doctor taking medical notes of an individual. They need to monitor the bipolar frequencies, the lengths as well as the individual's symptoms and their severity.

The Care and Treatments of someone who is Bipolar

Some of the best treatments available for someone with a Bipolar disorder may include a combination of medications and counseling. Some medications can include antipsychotic medications and lithium as well as "talk" sessions with a professional that specializes in this type of behavior.

Conclusions

A person that is diagnosed with a Bipolar Disorder needs to always remember that they can't tackle this medical condition on their own. They need a lot of support from their families, their friends as well as medical professionals. So after reading this self-help booklet, please seek the help that you may need to get your life back on track.

The End

This self-help booklet is a self-help guide that an individual could use to see if they may have some of the diagnoses or other symptoms listed in this book. This book also discusses some of the symptoms, treatments and testing procedures that may be used to diagnose an individual with this medical condition. A person must remember that they should not try and tackle this disease on their own, so please seek the medical help that you may need to get your life back on track if in fact you are diagnosed with this medical disorder.

Misty Lynn Wesley has a diversified career portfolio in the medical, legal, fashion and insurance industries. She is an avid blogger for Examiner, Yahoo Voices, and Helium. She also writes articles for CBS Local out of St. Paul, Minnesota and Believe.com on occasion. She has written four books with Publish America and several with Create Space which can be found on Amazon, Barnes and Noble and ITunes. She and her chosen producers have produced several audiobooks as well. So please feel free to check them out if you have the time. God bless.